-- for Beth, Bob, Joe, and Lorraine

Contents

A Word to the Wise…

And Everyone Else, Too!

It should be said that we – your authors Kelly and Ben – are neither doctors nor lawyers. Instead, we are senior living and memory care professionals with decades of experience under our belts. We can speak to trends and our own experiences, but your loved one is unique, and excellent care will reflect that uniqueness. There are no bulletproof solutions that will work universally, and compassion must always be combined with common sense to create loving, effective care.

You should always consult the appropriate professionals when caring for your loved one. If you have a medical question, nothing can substitute for the doctors and professionals who know your loved one's health history the best. If you have a legal question, talk to a lawyer. Always ask the appropriate expert to get the best results.

Introduction

First, thank you for taking the next step in supporting someone who is living with cognitive change. You're taking steps to manage and improve a difficult stage of your loved one's life, and that comes with a lot of conflicting feelings and difficult moments. You're not alone, and help is available. This guide will provide you with some key strategies for enriching your loved one's life and experiencing positive moments together.

For those of us caring for loved ones living with cognitive change, engaging them in daily life can be both difficult and rewarding. When it doesn't work, we might see the confusion in their eyes or watch them retreat into themselves. But when we get it right, when we draw them into an activity or conversation, we have given them an invitation to participate in the world for a time. These successful moments can be orchestrated, improved, and created reliably. Getting confident with engaging your loved one is what this guide is all about.

For caregivers of adults with dementia, understanding this evolution is crucial. Engagement, in its modern sense, highlights the importance of fostering deep connections and active participation in daily life. Engaging individuals with dementia in meaningful activities can significantly enhance their quality of life, providing them with a sense of purpose and involvement. By creating opportunities for them to participate in hobbies, social interactions, and physical activities, we honor the original spirit of engagement—commitment and connection—while adapting it to meet current needs. This approach not only helps in maintaining their cognitive functions but also brings joy and fulfillment to their lives, demonstrating that engagement is both essential and achievable.

Engagement is a vital part of everyone's day. It motivates us to get up in the morning, and it keeps us going throughout the day. If we fail to engage ourselves with rewarding work and favorite pastimes, we lose interest in the world around us. Especially for those living with cognitive change, it's crucial that they spend time with someone who understands what makes them feel fulfilled so that they can remain interested and active.

This book will provide ways to do just that. As you engage your loved one, you may just find yourself becoming more engaged too! In facilitating purpose for another, you will see your own sense of meaning flourish. In a difficult time, you may find ways to grow your relationship by rediscovering the commitment that bound you to that person in the first place. We hope these suggestions are helpful for you. Please send us your stories at elumened@elumened.com so we can all share in the hope.

Creating Purposeful Engagement

Book 1 in the
Cognitive Change Series

The Agreement: Meet Them Where They Are

Virtually all of the strategies we'll discuss at elumenEd assume that you are engaged in the agreement to "travel to them." This means that in order to calm, soothe, and engage loved ones, we must meet them where they are – and "where they are" may vary based on the time of day, the current need, their ability to ask for help, or the sensations they are having.

The journey to meet the person living with cognitive change can take many forms. You may have to pretend to be a different person, or live in a different time or place. You may have to find a way to let go of the fact that you've told them something 5 (or 50) times already. You may have to come to terms with their inability to perform a task they completed effortlessly in the past:

brushing their teeth, dressing themselves, or using simple objects around the house.

We know you're giving it all you've got, and you're amazing! Your loved one is also giving everything they have, and it can be hard to remember that sometimes. However, their reality is just as real for them as yours is for you. When, for instance, they look at you and see someone long-since passed, that is real for them. Let's take an imaginary "trip to them" and see how it might feel to walk in their shoes. Imagine if your spouse or child came home and insisted that they weren't your spouse or child. Can you imagine how unsettling that would be for you, even terrifying? And then what if your spouse, who says he's not your spouse, tells you that your actual spouse is dead? Or your child is dead? Or that you've lost your memory and your whole world isn't real? Would you believe them? How would you feel, learning every day for the first time, that your spouse of 50 years had passed away? That your child had died of breast cancer 15 years ago? It sounds to us like the worst possible waking nightmare, the stuff of horror movies, but it's also a situation that can be avoided with a little effort to meet your loved one in his or her reality. You can step into that reality and take on the roles they need you to take on. You can be that person's parent, or visit them in Paris, or reassure them that they are safe from a threat that they perceive. You are the ambassador to their world, bringing them comfort and compassion. When you meet them where they are, honoring and accepting their reality, you have a chance to see and interact with them at their most engaged.

This willingness to meet your loved one where he or she is at in this moment is the beginning of everything we will discuss.

Strategy #1: Asking for Advice and Opinions

Ask for advice or an opinion. This can be very empowering for your loved one, and may lead people with dementia to feel their wisdom matters. Keep the questions simple but meaningful.

As they tell stories, if they're lost in the story, you might simply listen quietly. Remember that sometimes asking the question is everything. It's ok to simply engage with your body language and attention: these are devices that allow all of us to feel heard in our daily lives. Your silence and attentiveness may give them space to talk.

On the other hand, if they are engaging with you, looking at you as they speak, and leaving silent spaces for you to talk, ask clarifying questions that prompt them to expand. Your goal will be to get them to engage in the storytelling process and keep them talking about their own life narrative. You can ask questions about things you want to know as well: family history, or that favorite recipe, or why Uncle Jeff hasn't talked to Aunt Sue for 47 years.

Remember, you don't need to correct them if you remember the story differently. We are going to their world, and honoring their memory is part of being their guest in that world. Allow them to tell their story, because it is true to them in this moment.

If they get to an event that agitates them, or they start getting upset because they can't remember part of their story, simply prompt or redirect them to a part of the story they enjoy. Try saying something like:

- Isn't that when... cousin Jeff moved back home to Uncle Gary and Aunt Virginia?

- That's too bad that happened, but what did you say about... that creative writing class in high school?
- It sounds like... dad was really handsome. Was he a good dancer?
- Would you tell me... about how you got through that?

Many of these are conversation tactics that we might use naturally with our peers, but it's difficult when dementia is involved because we may feel like it changes all of the rules.

We converse because we are social creatures and talking is how we are known. When we have someone we can confide in, we feel at peace. When we talk about our problems, joys, and worries, we feel known and loved. It can be challenging to find that comfortable space when we've had the same conversation over and over, or when our loved one's conversation doesn't remotely resemble the "real" world. However, can your commitment to that person create an environment where they feel heard and cared for? We believe that it can.

Here are some prompts you can use until you create your own:

Memories:

- "Can you tell me about where you grew up?"
- "What was your favorite thing to do as a child?"
- Family Traditions:
- "What holiday traditions did you have?"
- "Did you have any special family recipes?"
- School Days:
- "What subjects did you enjoy in school?"
- "Did you participate in any school activities or sports?"

Work and Career:"

- What was your first job?"
- "What are some memories from your favorite job?"

Favorite Activities:

- "What hobbies do you enjoy?"
- "What is your favorite trip you have ever taken? Tell me about it."

Books and Movies:
- "What is your favorite book or movie?"
- "What was your favorite story as a child?"

Music:
- "What kind of music do you enjoy?"
- "Who is your favorite singer or group?"
- "What is the best concert you've ever gone to?"

Everyday Life Daily Routines:
- "What is your favorite part of the day?"
- "How do you like to start/end your day?"

Meals and Cooking:
- "What is your favorite meal to cook or eat?"
- "Did you learn to cook from someone special?"

Pets and Animals:
- "Did you ever have a pet? Tell me about them."
- "What kind of animals do you like?"

Seasonal and Current Topics Holidays:

- "What is your favorite holiday memory?"
- "How did you usually celebrate holidays with your family?"

Current or Historical Events:

- "Did you hear about [a current event]? What do you think about it?"
- Name a significant moment in history and ask: "What were you doing when you found out?" Example: the day Kennedy was shot or the moon landing.

Visual and Sensory Prompts

- "Can you tell me the story behind this photo?"
- "Who is in this picture? What were you doing when it was taken?"
- "This [object] reminds me of something. Does it remind you of anything?"
- "What are some special items that mean a lot to you?" (offer examples such as a watch, awards)

General Prompts Favorites:

- "What is your favorite color/food/place?"
- "What is your favorite saying or quote?"

Opinions:

- "What do you think about [a general topic, like gardening, cooking, etc.]?"
- "Do you prefer [option A] or [option B]?"

Tips for Effective Communication

- Be Patient: Give them time to respond and don't rush the conversation.
- Offer prompts if they seem to be struggling.
- Ask Open Ended Questions rather than yes/no to encourage a response.
- Use Simple Language: Keep your questions and sentences straightforward.
- Be Encouraging: Show interest and enthusiasm in their responses.
- Listen Actively: Pay attention and respond to what they are saying.
- Avoid Correcting: Focus on the emotion behind their words rather than factual accuracy.

- Use Visual Aids: Photos, objects, and music can help spark memories and conversations.

Strategy #2: Do Some Chores

We all enjoy a grand adventure or a special activity: a trip to Greece, or maybe buying that car or dream home you've always wanted! Maybe it's a wedding or even having dinner at that swanky restaurant. But that's not what life is really made of. Those moments are exceptions to the rule.

The word "routine" comes from the Old French word "route," which we also, of course, still use. It meant then what it means now: a way, a path, a regular course, or a procedure. Our routines make up our lives: they are the path we travel each day. They can be counted on, we have control over them, and we spend our lives walking this routine day in and day out.

When we serve others, especially someone with dementia, our first response may be to try to lighten their load by taking away the burden of chores. It's meant to be a kindness, but we might actually be taking away that person's path in the process.

Instead, think of it like you would imagine life on the farm in the old days where everyone contributes to the family through their work and chores. On the farm, everyone receives appropriate tasks: you don't send a five-year-old to throw bales of hay! In the same way, you might not ask someone with dementia to use the stove or sharp knives. But what can they do? Your chore is to find ways that they can contribute, even if only in their own mind. Keep it safe and simple, and offer thanks and praise for their best efforts.

Here are some chores that might be appropriate for someone with different stages of memory loss. Choose the ones that fit your loved one, or come up with your own!

Simple Household Chores

Folding Laundry:

- Folding towels, clothes, or blankets can be a repetitive and soothing activity
- Sorting socks by color or matching pairs.

Setting the Table:

- Placing utensils/napkins/plates on the table.
- Arranging flowers or a centerpiece.

Dusting:

- Using a feather duster or a soft cloth to dust surfaces.
- Wiping down counters and tabletops.

Sweeping or Vacuuming:

- Sweeping small areas with broom and dustpan.
- Using a lightweight vacuum.

Watering Plants:

- Using a small watering can to water indoor or outdoor plants.
- Checking and misting plant leaves.

<u>**Kitchen-Related Chores:**</u>

Washing and Drying Dishes:

- Washing non-fragile dishes/utensils by hand.
- Drying dishes with a towel and putting them away.

Preparing Simple Meals:

- Peeling vegetables or fruit.
- Mixing ingredients for a salad or simple dish.
- Making sandwiches or snacks.

<u>**Grooming:**</u>

- Brushing their own hair.
- Selecting and laying out clothes for the day

<u>**Tidying Personal Space:**</u>

- Making the bed.
- Organizing personal items on a bedside table or dresser.

<u>**Outdoor Chores (supervised):**</u>

- Planting flowers or small plants.
- Weeding garden beds.
- Raking leaves into piles.
- Filling bird feeders.
- Placing birdseed in designated areas.

Sorting and Organizing:

- Sorting and organizing kitchen utensils.
- Arranging pantry items or groceries.
- Sorting buttons, coins, or other small items.
- Organizing photos or memorabilia.
- Sorting and organizing mail (with guidance).

Tips for Promoting Safety and Success

Supervision: Always supervise to ensure safety and provide assistance as needed.

Simplify Tasks: Break down tasks into manageable steps.

Use Familiar Tasks: Focus on chores they used to enjoy or are familiar with.

Provide Clear Instructions: Use simple, clear, and step-by-step instructions.

Create a Calm Environment: Ensure a quiet and distraction-free environment.

Be Patient: Allow them to work at their own pace and offer encouragement.

Ben's Story

My mom has felt a strong sense of purpose throughout her life because she sought out ways to help others. She grew up on a small dairy farm in the 50s and 60s, and "choring" was a way of life from before sun-up to after sun-down. It was how she understood her role in her family and her role in life. After graduating from a top music college, she started her teaching life sharing music with children in rural schools in Central New York. When she married my father, they started a print shop together where, again, they worked all day and weekends to make things work. Except for Sunday, that is, because my dad was a minister and she spent all day playing piano and tending to the "flock" as the "preacher's wife." My mother has led a very busy life of one chore after the next, building a life out of routine activities. Now that mom has dementia, she is taken care of so well that there aren't many chores to do. When we talk, she regularly mentions that she just wants to feel productive but she's not sure what to do. Living in a retirement community, she finds herself asking the concierge if she can help with paperwork. She wants to make her own bed and cook her own food. She wants to work and help others. More than watching TV or doing chair yoga, mom wants to do the chores that made up her first 80 years. Many memory care areas are not built to make this particularly easy, so how can you find ways? As an example, my mother is always kept well-supplied with yarn: she crochets like crazy and makes all sorts of things to donate. Now she's teaching other people at the community to crochet. These small chores and acts of service give her purpose.

Strategy #3: Incorporate Creative Expression

"Art washes away from the soul
the dust of everyday life."
-Pablo Picasso

How does creativity come to life in your world? Are you a musician or an artist? Are you learning a new computer program or building your social media audience? Do you act in a community theater? Maybe you like to blog or keep a journal. Perhaps a day can't go by without listening to your favorite musician or reading a chapter in a book.

For example, as we -- Kelly and Ben -- write this book, we feel purposeful. We feel like we're helping people and putting good things into the world. It's inspiring to have ideas, organize them, and share them with others who find value in what we're writing. This is our creative expression to share with the world, and that brings us a lot of joy and meaning.

Creative expression fuels that special part of the human spirit that wants to bring unique things into the world. No one else will ever paint like Picasso. No one else can write like William Faulkner or sing like Billie Holiday (or Billie Eilish!). Your care for your loved one is part of your creative expression: no one can care in the same way that you can. And no one can ever express themselves the way your loved one can. Dementia may alter this expression, but they're still a wholly unique person with the need to be known and to know others.

In the whole history of the universe, there has only ever been one of your loved one. He or she has never come before, and they will never come again. This life is their creative expression, and they are still expressing themselves. How can you tap into that and encourage it to help them create meaning?

The activities below provide some simple ways to create great impact by allowing for this expression and communication with the world. Where language fails, painting may succeed. Perhaps gardening or poetry will touch your loved one's soul after other memories have left. Try these activities and see what resonates with your loved one.

Ways to Incorporate Creative Expression:
Art Activities:
- Painting and Drawing: Use watercolors, acrylics, or colored pencils.
- Provide easy themes or let them draw freely.

Crafts:
- Engage in crafts like collages, clay modeling, or making decorations.

- Coloring Books: Provide adult coloring books with various themes.

Music:
- Listening: Play familiar songs or music from their past.
- Singing: Encourage them to sing along to their favorite tunes.
- Playing Instruments: If they played an instrument before, provide opportunities to play simple tunes.

Writing and Storytelling:
- Journaling: Encourage them to write about the day or their memories.
- Poetry: Read and/or write poems together.
- Storytelling: Share stories from their past or create new ones together.

Movement and Dance:
- Dancing: basic movements can be enjoyable and beneficial.

Gardening:

- Planting Flowers/Vegetables: Engage in small gardening tasks.
- Watering Plants: this repetitive task can provide a sense of purpose.

Prompts for Talking about Creative Expression: For Art Activities:

- "Would you like to try painting today? We can use some beautiful colors."
- "Let's make a collage together. We can use these magazines to find pictures we like."
- "Do you remember this song? It's one of your favorites. Let's listen to it together."
- "Would you like to sing along with me? We can sing some of the songs you love."
- "How about writing a little about what we did today? It could be fun to look back on later."
- "Can you tell me a story from when you were young? I love hearing your stories."
- "Shall we dance a little? We can move to the rhythm of this music."

- "Let's do some gentle exercises together. It will be fun and good for us."
- "Would you like to help me water the plants? They always look so happy after a drink."
- "Let's plant some flowers today. It's so rewarding to watch them grow."

Tips for Facilitating Creativity:
- Be Patient and Gentle: Approach them with patience and a calm demeanor.
- Use Simple Language: Keep sentences short and clear.
- Offer Choices: Give them options to choose from to encourage participation.
- Focus on Enjoyment: Emphasize the fun and relaxing aspects rather than the outcome.
- Be Encouraging: Praise their efforts and participation, regardless of the results.

Strategy #4: Exercise

Exercise is widely recognized as beneficial for overall brain health and may help slow the progression of Alzheimer's disease. It doesn't stop the disease – nothing we've discovered yet can – but regular physical activity can have several positive effects that might slow the progression of symptoms. Everyone responds in their own unique way, but exercise is beneficial for all and might positively impact both your loved one's body and mind. Some of the amazing benefits of exercise for people living with dementia include:

- **Neurogenesis:** Physical activity promotes neurogenesis, the formation of new neurons, particularly in the hippocampus, an area of the brain crucial for memory.
- **Synaptic Plasticity:** Exercise enhances synaptic plasticity, which is the ability of synapses (connections between neurons) to strengthen or weaken over time, in

response to increases or decreases in their activity. This is essential for learning and memory.

- **Reduction of Beta-Amyloid:** Regular physical activity has been shown to reduce the accumulation of beta-amyloid plaques, which are characteristic of Alzheimer's disease and contribute to the death of brain cells.
- **Anti-Inflammatory Effects:** Exercise has anti-inflammatory effects, reducing chronic inflammation in the brain that is associated with Alzheimer's disease.
- **Increased Levels of Brain-Derived Neurotrophic Factor (BDNF):** BDNF is a protein that supports the survival, development, and function of neurons. Exercise increases BDNF levels, which helps in maintaining and forming new connections in the brain.

All of this may lead to improved moods and stress reduction. We want to emphasize that exercise isn't a magic bullet. But there can be shifts, sometimes significant shifts, when you encourage your loved one to engage their brain/body connection.

We've listed some possible exercises below, but please keep in mind that exercises must be selected and tailored to each person's capabilities. Start slowly: you're not trying to help your loved one run a marathon. The goal is to facilitate simple movement that keeps the brain firing those signals to the body so he or she can stay mobile and retain musculature.

> *Always check with your loved one's physician before starting an exercise routine.*

Gentle Aerobic Exercises

- **Walking:** Make sure footwear is appropriate and that walking surfaces are free from cracks in the sidewalk or other trip hazards.

- **Swimming:** Swimming or water aerobics are gentle on the joints and can be very soothing. For seniors who have been swimmers throughout their lives, this may be an excellent exercise that brings back past moments and activates muscle memory.

- **Stationary Bicycling:** Using a stationary bike can improve cardiovascular health without the risk of falling. Take it nice and slow. Many bikes and other aerobic exercise machines now have heart monitoring capabilities that you can take advantage of as well.

Flexibility and Balance

- **Tai Chi:** Tai Chi is a slow and gentle form of exercise that can improve balance, coordination, and reduce stress. If you go this route, make sure you find a qualified instructor who understands the special needs of seniors with dementia. Consider reaching out to a local memory care provider for recommendations.

- **Yoga:** Simple yoga poses and breathing exercises enhance flexibility, balance, and relaxation. Chair yoga is a good option for those with limited mobility. Again, look for a qualified yoga instructor who understands your loved one's special needs. Contacting a memory care provider can, once again, be a great way to find a qualified instructor.

Tips for Exercising with Alzheimer's Disease

- **Consistency:** Try to incorporate exercise into a daily routine.
- **Supervision:** Ensure someone is present to provide support and ensure safety.
- **Adaptability:** Be ready to modify exercises based on the person's abilities and preferences.
- **Enjoyment:** Choose activities the person enjoys to keep them motivated.

- **Comfort:** Ensure they are wearing comfortable clothing and proper footwear.
- **Hydration:** Make sure they drink plenty of water before, during, and after exercise.
- **Duration:** Aim for short sessions (10-30 minutes) to avoid fatigue.

Remember that exercise for a senior with dementia doesn't mean a 60-minute sweat-drenched workout. It might just be a walk across the house and back, or practicing the first three moves in a Tai Chi form for a couple of minutes. Small steps (literally) can make for big results. Take it slow and be encouraging.

Strategy #5: Get Back to Nature

*In every walk with nature
one receives far more than he seeks.*
-John Muir

There is something special in nature, from gardening in the backyard to visiting the Grand Canyon to climbing Mount Everest, most of us find ourselves when we return to the vastness of the earth we live in. Nature is a vital component of overall well being for all of us. When our loved ones can be outside for even short bursts, weather permitting, they may experience a lessening of agitation and a sense of peace.

A caveat: someone with cognitive change should <u>never</u> be left unattended outdoors and should be monitored for comfort when outside. They may wander away and get lost, or they may be exposed to heat or cold and not realize they need to go inside, hydrate, or put on heavier clothing. This can create a lethal situation. However, with monitoring, a trip into nature can be a healing experience and a joyful time.

Getting in Touch with Nature

Walking

- Nature Walks
- Guided Tours of botanical gardens, arboretums, or nature reserves

Gardening

- Planting Flowers
- Watering Plants
- Weeding and Pruning

Bird Watching

- Feeding Birds
- Using Binoculars to find local birds

Nature Crafts

- Collecting Natural Items like leaves, flowers, or rocks
- Painting or decorating rocks

Strategy #6: Music is Magic

"Music expresses that which cannot be put into words and that which cannot remain silent."
— *Victor Hugo*

Music is magic! Using music that is specific to your loved one's life history can be a great mood elevator and might even make for an impromptu dance party in the living room! Music can transport our loved ones back in time: to moments of spiritual peace through hymns sung in a childhood church, or to Woodstock with Jimmy Hendrix, or to the Jazz Showcase club in Chicago with Herbie Hancock. Music moves us through time and place like few other things can, as every shower karaoke master can attest! So how can you tap into this?

Take advantage of technology:

- Use an app like Spotify or YouTube Music to create a playlist of music that has played an important role in your loved one's life and use this to motivate, entertain, and soothe.

- Use a bluetooth-enabled speaker to amplify the volume: your phone may not be loud enough if your loved one has any hearing difficulty.

- You can make different lists of different genres of music and discern what your person is in the mood for today.

> Pro-tip: give them just two different genres of music from which to choose. More than that might be confusing.

- Get creative about the different places where you play music with them. It doesn't have to just be at home, especially with an app on your phone that, thanks to the internet, can access virtually any music in the world in most places that you will be.

Can they be a music maker?

- Is your loved one a musician? Is there a way that they can still make music? You might be surprised at how, when other tasks seem too complicated, the brain-body connection and muscle memory will still combine to allow people to create music. Some instruments, particularly string instruments and pianos, have headphone jacks that will prevent the noise from being heard by others.

What stories can they tell about the music they love?

- Talk to them. Ask questions. What's their favorite song? Artist?
- Did they have a favorite concert they went to? What was that like?
- Did they sing their children any favorite lullaby songs? (If you are their adult child, perhaps you could sing them together.)

- Is there a song that has a special meaning to them or reminds them of a significant moment in their lives?
- Was there a special song that they shared with their partner as "their song"?

Kelly's Story

A move to a memory care program can be a difficult transition. For a resident we'll call "Ellen," it was a particularly confusing time. To make the community a more familiar place, her family donated Ellen's beloved grand piano to the community, something she enjoyed playing daily at home. Ellen didn't remember the piano was hers and she couldn't read music any longer, but she could play from memory beautifully. It is thought that the reason this is possible is that the regions of the brain responsible for music memory, such as the cerebellum, may not be affected until later in the disease. This makes music such a powerful way to reach someone when other mechanisms fail. Just as music touches a special place in the heart, it also touches a special place in the mind that allows people with dementia to access memories and emotions even after other stimuli are no longer as effective.

Ben's story

My mother had been living in an independent setting for about a year, but she made the transition to Assisted Living after dementia started taking a difficult toll. It was challenging for both of us and, despite making a great go of things, she struggled to find her place and purpose in the new environment over the first couple of weeks.

The Housekeeping Director in the building is aware that my mom has a musical background. Mom was classically trained as a flautist (a fancy word for flute player) at the prestigious Crane School of Music in Potsdam, NY; worked as a music teacher; and spent much of her life playing piano at the churches where my late father was the minister.

Music would soothe her and nourish her spirit. We weren't sure what to do to fulfill this need in the assisted environment, however. Knowing this, that director brought in a keyboard that she wasn't using and gifted it to my mother. Mom can now play piano in her apartment, but it's also light enough that it can be brought out to play for other residents as well. Headphones with with the keyboard as well, so we won't disturb her neighbors during the sessions that come later in the evening.

Another employee is a fellow piano player, and they played songs together and traded notes. Mom told these two employees that "Something was missing in my soul, and this fills it." I think that says it all. I will always be grateful to them for their generosity and compassion.

Afterword:

Looking through the Lens of Possibility

What you're going through, and what Kelly and Ben are going through with their parents too, is not fair. There is no dancing around that fact: you are suffering, your loved one is suffering, and it's terrible. No amount of sugar coating or pretending or pity from friends will ever make it better. Dementia is terrible for everyone involved. We can't change the truth of that. None of us can.

However, the strategies we talked about throughout this guide may allow you to make a small but important shift: a shift in perspective. When we look into the face of dementia day after day, the "can'ts" start to pile up. Eventually, that might be all we can see anymore:

You can't go outside by yourself.

You can't eat that.

You can't use the stove.

You can't drive the car.

You can't have your credit card.

You can't use breakable plates.

You can't go to the bathroom by yourself.

You can't...

On and on: you can't. And of course, those "can'ts" matter. They help to keep our loved ones safe. But what if we looked at things in a different way when we're looking for redirections? What if we started looking at the same situation and seeing the "cans"? What if we started looking at the possibilities rather than the impracticalities? What if we stopped looking for scarcity and started looking for abundance?

The parable below demonstrates the principle nicely. What happens when two people see the same situation with different viewpoints, scarcity

"A shoe factory sends two marketing scouts to a region of Africa to study the prospects for expanding the business. One sends back a telegram saying,

"SITUATION HOPELESS STOP
NO ONE WEARS SHOES

"The other writes back triumphantly,

"GLORIOUS BUSINESS OPPORTUNITY STOP THEY HAVE NO SHOES"

-*The Art of Possibility,*
Rosamund Stone Zander and Benjamin Zander

The activities in this guide give you the tools you need to view interactions with your loved one through the lens of abundance. The Roman philosopher Cicero is credited with the saying, "Where there is life, there is hope."

There is still life, and there is hope today, for you and your loved one. There is an opportunity to connect with each other, to engage with activities, and to be the person you want to be in the face of a difficult situation. There is hope for your loved one to shine through for a moment, to smile, to enjoy a favorite song, to leave agitation and worry behind for an instant.

We hope this guide provides you with hope, abundance, and many possibilities. Please feel free to contact us at elumened@elumened.com to share your stories and feedback. Good luck to you in this difficult endeavor. You are not alone.

"We are all in this together. We are each of us angels with only one wing, and we can only fly by embracing one another."

-Luciano De Crescenzo

About the Authors

Ben Couch

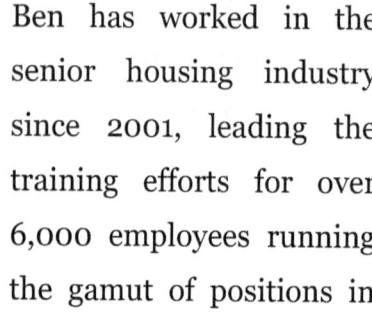

Ben has worked in the senior housing industry since 2001, leading the training efforts for over 6,000 employees running the gamut of positions in As an educational leader, he has spent decades working with experts in cognitive change to create pragmatic, compassionate care programs for seniors living with dementia. As his mother now moves through the stages of Alzheimer's disease, his vocation has taken on new meaning as the principles discussed in this book have become his own personal lifelines.

Kelly Ording

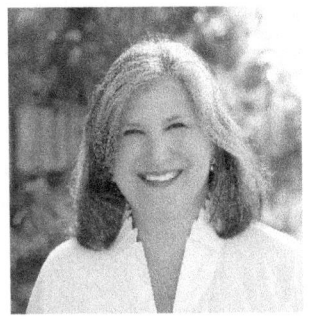

Kelly is a passionate advocate for adults living with dementia. Having spent her career as a champion of people living with dementia, she believes that we can improve the lives of those we serve through training the individuals who serve them. As a trainer for SAGE (Services and Advocacy for LGBTQ+ Elders) and the National Council of Certified Dementia Practitioners, she has trained hundreds of caregivers across the country.

www.ingramcontent.com/pod-product-compliance
Lightning Source LLC
Chambersburg PA
CBHW070136230526
45472CB00004B/1552